LILA GLOWSTONE

Skin Deep: Unlocking the Secrets to Radiant Skin

A Guide to Skin Types, Skincare Ingredients and Creating Your Own Routines for Radiant Skin

Copyright © 2024 by Lila Glowstone

All rights reserved. No part of this publication may be reproduced, stored or transmitted in any form or by any means, electronic, mechanical, photocopying, recording, scanning, or otherwise without written permission from the publisher. It is illegal to copy this book, post it to a website, or distribute it by any other means without permission.

This novel is entirely a work of fiction. The names, characters and incidents portrayed in it are the work of the author's imagination. Any resemblance to actual persons, living or dead, events or localities is entirely coincidental.

Lila Glowstone asserts the moral right to be identified as the author of this work.

Lila Glowstone has no responsibility for the persistence or accuracy of URLs for external or third-party Internet Websites referred to in this publication and does not guarantee that any content on such Websites is, or will remain, accurate or appropriate.

Designations used by companies to distinguish their products are often claimed as trademarks. All brand names and product names used in this book and on its cover are trade names, service marks, trademarks and registered trademarks of their respective owners. The publishers and the book are not associated with any product or vendor mentioned in this book. None of the companies referenced within the book have endorsed the book.

First edition

This book was professionally typeset on Reedsy.
Find out more at reedsy.com

Contents

1

Introduction

Welcome to the world of skincare where the search for perfect skin is always on. With so many products, routines and advice out there, it's no wonder it can feel like the perfect complexion is an impossible task. But fear not, this guide will get to the bottom of radiant skin and help you make sense of the skincare chaos.

Skin Deep: Get the Glow is your guide to skin types, skincare ingredients and creating your own routines for glowing skin. This book is not just about surface level beauty but about understanding the importance of skincare for overall health and well-being.

Our skin is the largest organ of our body and plays a vital role in protecting us from the outside world. Yet we often neglect to give it the care and attention it needs. Skin Deep will take you on a journey to get to the inside out of healthy and glowing skin.

In this book you'll learn about the different skin types and how to figure out yours. You'll get to the bottom of the science behind skincare ingredients and how they work to improve your skin. With this knowledge you'll be able to create your own skincare routine that's tailored to your needs and concerns.

No more following beauty trends and using products that may not be suitable for your skin. Skin Deep will give you the information and tools to make informed decisions and take control of your skincare journey. With the right knowledge and products, healthy and glowing skin is within your grasp.

So, are you ready to get the glow? Let Skin Deep be your guide on this journey to a healthier and more beautiful you. Say goodbye to dull and lifeless skin and hello to a radiant complexion that shines from within.

Let's get started and discover the power of healthy skin.

Chapter 1: Understanding Your Skin

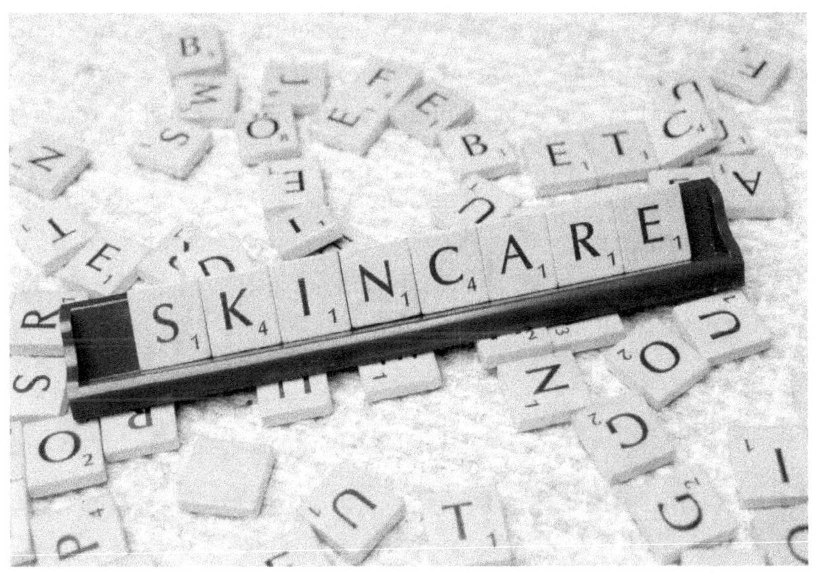

S kin health is often overlooked in our daily lives as we are constantly bombarded with ads for the latest makeup and beauty products. But we must remember that our skin is not just a canvas for us to paint on but it's an organ that is our body's first line of defense against the outside world. Our skin protects us from UV rays, bacteria and other environmental factors that can harm our overall health. So, we must prioritize and take care of our skin health.

Healthy skin not only protects us physically but also plays a crucial role in our self esteem and confidence. Our skin is a reflection of our inner health and when it's well nourished and taken care of, it can give us a radiant glow. On the other hand, neglecting our skin can lead to skin issues like acne, dryness, premature aging and even serious conditions like skin cancer.

Besides physical and mental health, skin health also affects our overall health. Our skin regulates our body temperature, absorbs nutrients and eliminates toxins. When our skin is unhealthy it can disrupt these functions and lead to a weak immune system and other health problems.

So, skin health matters for not just our physical appearance but for our overall health and overall well-being. Let's not neglect this vital organ and make an effort to take care of our skin not just for its aesthetic value but for our overall health and happiness.

Skin Types Demystified

Identifying Your Skin Type

To care for your skin, you first need to know it. Like a symphony, your skin works in layers to protect, heal and communicate with the rest of your body. The first step in this journey is to identify your skin type. Imagine trying to solve a puzzle without seeing the final picture; that's what it's like using skincare products without knowing your skin. Skin types generally fall into 5 categories: dry, oily, combination, sensitive and normal.

In our daily routine we often forget to pay attention to our skin. We take our skin for granted, assuming it will always be there to protect us. But have you ever stopped to really know your skin and all that it does for you?

One of the most important things to know about your skin is that it's unique to you. Just like your fingerprints, no two people have the same skin. Your skin type is determined by a combination of genetics and environmental factors. That's why what works for your friend's skin may not necessarily work for yours.

In order to determine your skin type, observe your skin throughout the day. Does it get shiny by noon or does it feel dry and tight? A simple test is to wash your face with a gentle cleanser, wait for an hour and then check your skin. This is the foundation upon which you can build your skincare routine, so every product you use addresses your skin's needs.

Not all skin is created equal. Your skin's behavior is determined by genetics, lifestyle and even the weather. Here's how to determine your skin type:

Dry Skin

- Lacks moisture, dry skin often feels tight especially after washing. It may also look dull or flaky.
- Example: During winter, Emma's cheeks felt rough and started

peeling—a sign her skin needed more hydration.

Oily Skin

- Produces excess sebum, causes shine, enlarged pores and a tendency towards acne.
- Solution: Use non-comedogenic products to not clog pores further.

Combination Skin

- A mix of oily and dry areas, usually with oily T-zone (forehead, nose and chin) and dry cheeks.
- Tip: Use light products on oily areas and richer creams on dry areas.

Sensitive Skin

- Prone to redness, irritation or stinging.
- Advice: Always patch test new products and avoid known irritants like alcohol and synthetic fragrances.

Normal Skin

- Balanced and low maintenance, normal skin doesn't break out or react to products.
- Example: Alex's skin stays smooth and comfortable even after trying new products, that's a healthy skin barrier.

DIY Skin Test: Wash your face, wait an hour and press a tissue to your skin.

- **Dry:** No oil on the tissue.
- **Oily:** Oil on all areas.
- **Combination:** Oil on T-zone only.

The Science of Skin Structure and Function

In addition to your skin type, you should also know the layers of your skin. Your skin has three main layers, each has its own function:

Epidermis: Your Protective Shield

- This topmost layer is a barrier against environmental stressors like pollution, bacteria and harmful UV rays. It also regulates water loss.
- It's made up of keratinocytes which produce keratin—a protein that's important for skin strength. The outermost part, stratum corneum, is made up of dead cells that shed naturally.
- Example: If your skin feels rough, it's probably because of the buildup of dead cells, time to exfoliate.

Dermis: The Skin's Command Center

- Beneath the epidermis is the dermis where everything happens. This layer is where collagen (for structure), elastin (for elasticity) and hyaluronic acid (for hydration) are found.
- It also has blood vessels that nourish the skin and nerve endings that allow you to feel sensations.

Hypodermis: The Insulating Layer

- The hypodermis is made up of fat, it's the cushioning and temperature regulator.
- Did You Know? This layer also stores energy in the form of fat.

Analogy: Think of your skin like a well-built house. The epidermis is the roof, shielding the house from rain and sun. The dermis is the framework, providing structure and functionality, while the hypodermis is the foundation, keeping everything stable.

Skin Conditions and Concerns

With all the skin types and conditions out there, it can be confusing to know what your skin needs. That's why you should know the common skin conditions and concerns like acne, hyperpigmentation and aging and how to address them effectively.

Acne

Acne occurs when hair follicles (pores) get clogged with oil (sebum), dead skin cells and sometimes bacteria. This can lead to:

- **Blackheads:** Open clogged pores where the surface turns dark due to oxidation.
- **Whiteheads:** Closed clogged pores with trapped oil and dead skin.
- **Pimples:** Inflamed red bumps caused by bacteria or irritation in clogged pores.

Causes:

- **Excess Sebum Production:** Often linked to hormonal changes (puberty, menstruation, pregnancy).
- **Bacteria:** Propionibacterium acnes (P. acnes) thrive in clogged pores, causing inflammation.
- **Lifestyle Factors:** Diet (high in dairy, sugar), stress and poor skincare.
- **Genetics:** Family history of acne increases risk.

Treatment Options:

Topical Treatments:

- **Salicylic Acid:** Exfoliates inside the pores to clear and prevent clogs.
- **Benzoyl Peroxide:** Kills acne-causing bacteria.
- **Retinoids:** Unclog pores and promote cell turnover.

Oral Medications:

- Antibiotics, hormonal treatments (like birth control), or isotretinoin for severe cases.

Lifestyle Adjustments:

- Cleanse skin gently, don't over scrub.
- Eat a balanced diet and reduce stress.

Hyperpigmentation

Hyperpigmentation occurs when the skin produces excess melanin and creates dark spots or patches. It can appear in areas exposed to the sun but can also appear anywhere.

Causes:

- **Sun Exposure:** UV rays trigger melanin production as a response to protect the skin and create dark patches over time.
- **Hormonal Changes:** Pregnancy or conditions like melasma can cause hormone induced pigmentation.
- Post-Inflammatory Hyperpigmentation (PIH): Dark spots after acne, injuries or other skin trauma.
- **Medications:** Some drugs like chemotherapy agents or birth control can stimulate melanin production.

Treatment Options:

Topical Treatments:

- **Vitamin C:** Brightens skin and reduces melanin production.
- **Hydroquinone:** Lightens dark patches (short term use only).
- **Niacinamide:** Reduces pigmentation and strengthens the skin barrier.
- **AHAs/BHAs:** Chemical exfoliants like glycolic acid clears out dead skin cells and fades dark spots.

Professional Procedures:

- **Chemical Peels**: Deeper exfoliation to target stubborn pigmentation.
- **Laser Treatments:** Breaks down excess melanin for even skin tone.
- **Prevention:** Always wear sunscreen (SPF 30+) to prevent further pigmentation and darkening of existing spots.

Aging

Skin aging is a natural process where structural proteins like collagen and elastin decline and cause wrinkles, fine lines and sagging. Other signs are dryness, dullness and thinner skin.

Causes:

- **Intrinsic Aging:** Natural decline in skin elasticity and hydration due to age.
- **Extrinsic Aging:** Environmental factors like UV exposure, pollution and lifestyle habits speed up the process.
- **Loss of Fat and Bone Density:** Causes hollowness and skin sagging.
- **Slower Cell Turnover:** Results to rough texture and uneven tone.

Treatment Options:

Topical Treatments:

- **Retinoids:** Stimulates collagen production and improves texture.
- **Peptides:** Signals the skin to repair and rebuild collagen.
- **Antioxidants:** Protects against free radical damage (e.g., vitamin

C, E and ferulic acid).
- Hyaluronic Acid: Plumps and hydrates to minimize fine lines.

Professional Procedures:

- Microneedling: Stimulates collagen production.
- Dermal Fillers: Fills up lost volume in sagging areas.
- Botox: Reduces dynamic wrinkles caused by repetitive muscle movement.

Prevention:

- Wear sunscreen daily to slow down UV induced aging.
- Live a healthy lifestyle (balanced diet, no smoking and regular hydration).

Having any of these skin conditions can be frustrating and even affect our self esteem. But the good news is, with the right skincare routine and products, acne can be managed and even prevented. Look for products that have salicylic acid or benzoyl peroxide which can unclog pores and reduce inflammation. Also, make sure to wash your face twice a day and don't touch your face with your hands to prevent further breakouts.

To address hyperpigmentation, it is important to protect your skin from the sun. Wear sunscreen daily and use products with brightening ingredients like vitamin C and niacinamide. Consistency is key when it comes to treating hyperpigmentation so be patient and stick to your routine for best results.

As we age, our skin also goes through changes. Collagen and elastin which are responsible for keeping our skin firm and supple declines and causes wrinkles and fine lines. While aging is a natural process, there are ways to slow it down and look youthful. Incorporate anti-aging products in our skincare routine such as retinoids, hyaluronic acid and peptides to stimulate collagen production and improve overall skin tone.

Aside from these common skin conditions, there are other concerns that may affect our skin such as dryness, sensitivity and redness. Listen to your skin and be aware of any changes or reactions. If you have sensitive skin, go for gentle and fragrance-free products. For dry skin, look for hydrating ingredients like ceramides and glycerin. And if you experience redness or irritation, products with soothing ingredients like aloe vera or chamomile can calm and heal your skin.

So, there you have it, understanding your skin and its needs is the key to healthy and glowing skin. Don't be afraid to try and find what works for you. Be patient and consistent with your skincare routine and consult a dermatologist if you have any concerns. With the right information and approach, you can conquer any skin condition or concern and feel good in your own skin. Start taking care of your skin now and see the difference it can make to your overall well-being.

3

Chapter 4: Beyond Skincare

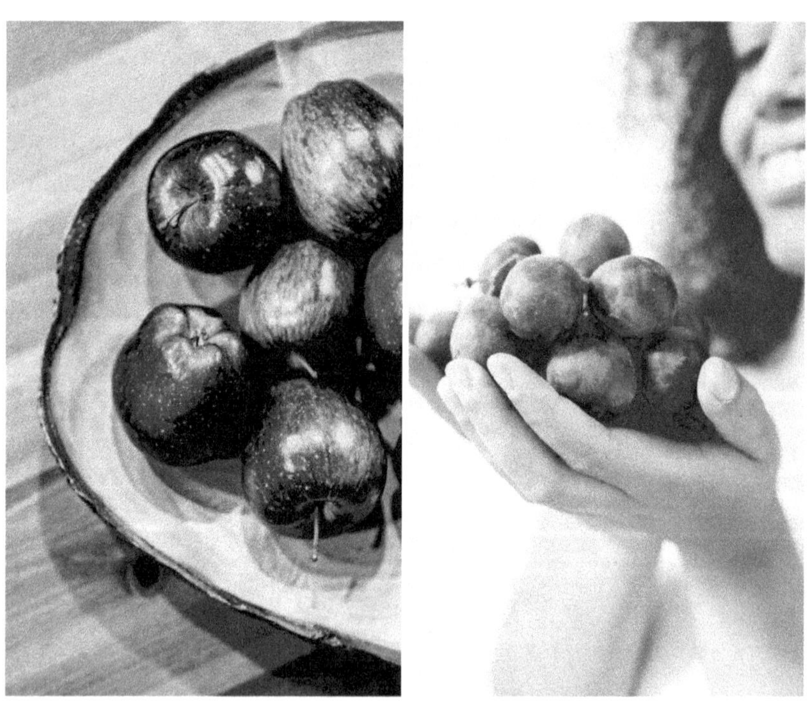

As we go through our daily lives, we often forget what we put into our bodies. We are bombarded with ads for expensive skincare products that promise a radiant and flawless complexion but the truth is, the key to having healthy and glowing skin starts from within. The role of diet and nutrition in achieving beautiful skin is often overlooked but it's a crucial factor that should not be ignored.

What we eat affects our skin. Eating a diet rich in whole, unprocessed foods like fruits, vegetables, whole grains and lean proteins gives our skin the vitamins and minerals it needs to stay healthy. These nutrients help repair damaged skin cells, promote collagen production and maintain a youthful look.

On the other hand, a diet rich in processed foods, sugar and unhealthy fats can cause inflammation in the body which can manifest on our skin as acne, eczema and premature aging. These foods also lack the nutrients our skin needs making it dull, dry and prone to breakouts.

In a world where beauty standards are as diverse as the stars in the sky, the pursuit of glowing skin feels like chasing a mirage. Yet, the secret to radiant skin is not just in the creams and serums we apply but in a holistic approach that includes mind, body and spirit. This story goes beyond skincare where beauty is not just skin deep but a reflection of overall wellness.

Think of beauty as a tapestry, woven with threads of physical health, mental clarity and emotional balance. This holistic approach to beauty is gaining popularity as more people realize that true radiance comes from within. It's about nourishing the body with healthy foods, exercising regularly and having a positive mindset.

Diet and Hydration

The saying "you are what you eat" is especially true when it comes to skin health. There are foods that have been proven to have specific benefits for our skin. A diet rich in:

- **Antioxidant-Rich Foods:** Include spinach, blueberries and green tea to combat oxidative stress. They help protect our skin from free radical damage and slow down the aging process.
- **Hydration:** Drink at least 8 glasses of water daily and eat hydrating foods like watermelon. Hydration is a key to radiant skin. Drinking water throughout the day flushes out toxins from our body and keeps our skin hydrated, plump and glowing. Dehydration on the other hand makes our skin look dull and dry.

Also worth noting is that certain dietary habits like smoking and excessive alcohol consumption can harm our skin. These habits can cause premature aging, dehydration and dullness.

Stress Management

Chronic stress raises cortisol, a hormone that can cause breakouts and redness. In the chaos of modern life, stress gets to our skin. Cortisol, the stress hormone, can trigger inflammation and worsen conditions like acne and eczema. Mindfulness practices like meditation and yoga are a sanctuary for the mind, reducing stress and promoting skin health.

Beyond diet and mindfulness, other lifestyle habits play a big role in achieving and maintaining beautiful skin. Regular exercise for example boosts circulation, delivering oxygen and nutrients to skin cells. It also promotes collagen production, the protein that keeps skin firm and youthful.

Also, enough sleep is necessary for skin regeneration. During deep sleep, the body repairs damaged cells and produces new ones resulting in fresher looking skin. Prioritizing sleep hygiene like having a consistent sleep schedule and creating a sleep conducive environment can boost your skin's vitality.

For example, a study in Journal of Clinical and Aesthetic Dermatology found that green tea extract can reduce sebum production and improve acne symptoms. By choosing products with natural ingredients, you can minimize exposure to harsh chemicals and support your skin's natural healing.

4

Chapter 2: The Science of Skincare Ingredients

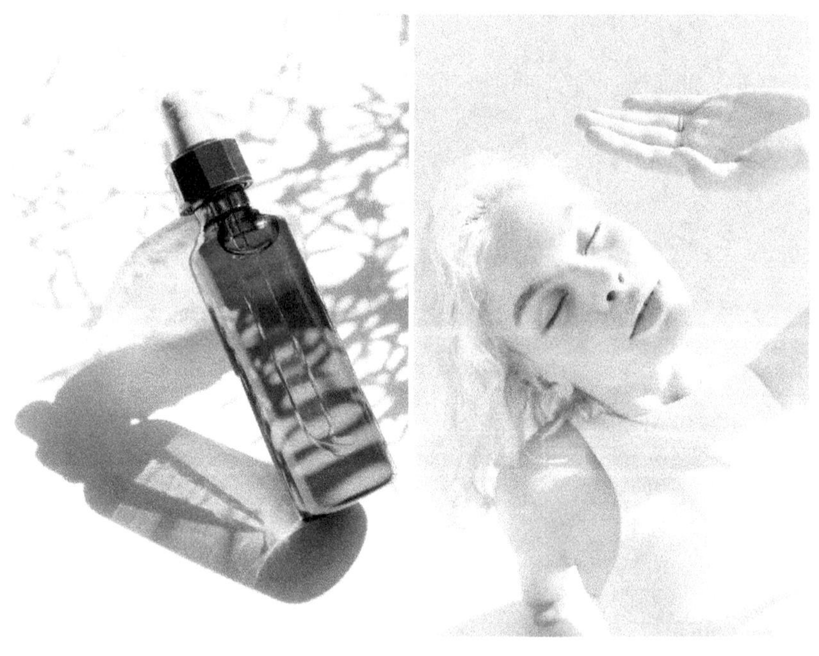

I n the world of skincare where promises of perfect skin are as common as the sunrise, understanding the science behind skincare ingredients is like finding the golden ticket. The journey to glowing skin is not just about applying the latest cream or serum; it's about knowing what's in these products and how they work with your skin.

Once you've determined your skin type, the next step is to understand the science behind skincare ingredients. This is like the ingredients in a recipe—they determine if the final result will be a feast for your skin or a disaster. Each one has a specific role like the players in an orchestra working together to create harmony.

But not all ingredients are for all skin types. Let's get into it.

Decoding Ingredient Labels

Read product labels and know what each ingredient does. This will empower you to make informed decisions and choose products that will improve your skin and not worsen existing concerns. So learning to read labels will save you from using ineffective or harmful products.

Power Players - Key Ingredients and Their Benefits

Imagine unlocking your skincare routine with ingredients that really work on your skin. It's not just about products; it's about choosing the right ingredients that work with your skin's natural processes.

Let's get into some of the power players:

Hyaluronic Acid

- The hydration hero. Can hold up to 1,000 times its weight in water, this super molecule quenches your skin's thirst, leaves it plump, smooth and glowing. It's the ultimate solution for dryness and fine lines.
- Example: Apply after cleansing and before moisturizing for a glowing skin.

Vitamin C

- The glow-giver. Packed with antioxidants, it brightens dull skin, fades dark spots and protects against environmental stressors like pollution and UV rays. With regular use, Vitamin C will make your skin look like it's lit from within.
- Pro Tip: Look for stable formulations like magnesium ascorbyl phosphate to avoid oxidation.

Retinoids

- The gold standard in anti-aging. This powerful derivative of Vitamin A increases collagen production, smooths wrinkle and accelerates cell turnover for visibly new skin. It's like giving your skin a daily reboot.
- Example: Start slow to minimize irritation, use retinol once or twice a week to begin with.

Niacinamide

- A multi-tasking wonder. Minimizes pores, balances oil production and strengthens the skin barrier. Whether you're fighting acne, redness or uneven tone, niacinamide works gently but effectively to restore balance to your skin
- Tip: Use niacinamide with hyaluronic acid for a soothing, hydrating combo.

Salicylic Acid

- A blemish-fighting superhero. For acne-prone skin, it goes deep into the pores to dissolve excess oil and unclog buildup. The result? Clearer, healthier skin that feels as good as it looks.
- Tip: Start using it 2-3 times a week to let your skin adjust, especially if you have sensitive skin

Ingredients to Avoid

- Sulfates: Found in foaming cleansers, they strip natural oils and cause irritation.
- Synthetic Fragrances: Found in high-end products but a major irritant for sensitive skin

Each of these ingredients has its own role to play in the skin of your dreams. The key is to know your skin and choose the right combination. Choose wisely and let your skin show off its best—because the right ingredients can make all the difference.

Now that we know about ingredients, it's also important to understand how they work together. Skincare products are formulated with specific combinations of ingredients to address different skin concerns. For example, if you have oily skin, you would look for products with ingredients like salicylic acid or tea tree oil that helps control oil production and prevent breakouts.

In addition to knowing ingredients, it's also important to know how to use skincare products. Many people make the mistake of using too many products or not using them in the right order and it can cause adverse effects on the skin. Follow the recommended usage and application instructions for each product to get the best results.

In a nutshell, the science of skincare ingredients is crucial to having healthy and glowing skin. Educate yourself on what ingredients are good and bad and how they work together to address different skin concerns. By understanding the science behind skincare, we can make informed decisions on the products we use and get the best for our skin. So next time you're shopping for skincare products, take a closer look at the ingredients and choose wisely for your skin's sake.

5

Chapter 3: Your Skincare Routine

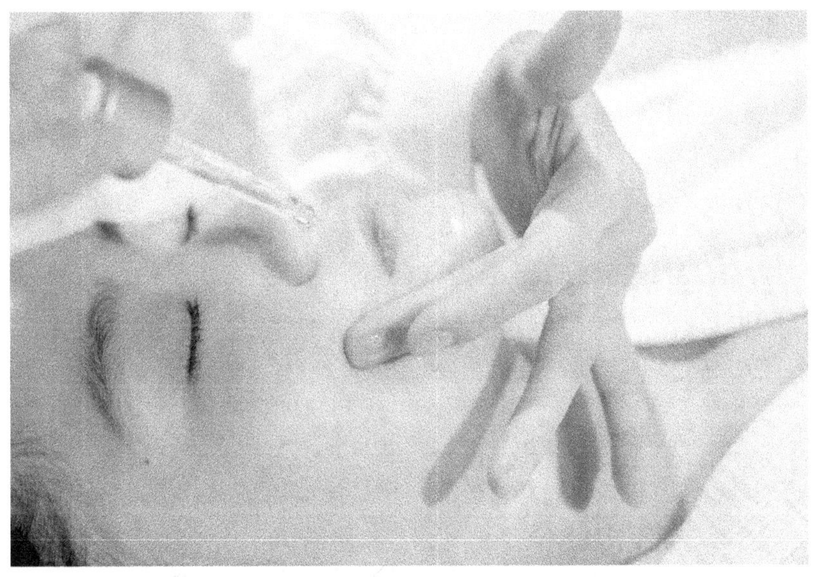

Creating your own skincare routine is key to having healthy and glowing skin. Every skin is unique and what works for one may not work for another. So it's important to know your skin type and its needs to create a routine that addresses its individual requirements.

Once you know your skin type, the next step is to determine your skin concerns. Do you have acne, fine lines, dark spots, uneven texture? These concerns will guide you in choosing the right products and treatments to address them.

Now that you know your skin type and the science of skincare ingredients, it's time to create your own skincare routine. Think of this routine as a bespoke suit, made to fit your skin perfectly. A basic routine includes:

Morning Routine

Cleanse

- Why: At night, your skin produces sweat, oil and may collect dust or debris from your pillowcase. Cleansing gives you a fresh start for the day.
- How to Use: Wet your face with lukewarm water, apply a gentle cleanser for your skin type and massage in circular motions. Rinse thoroughly and pat dry with a clean towel.
- Tips: Don't use harsh cleansers that strip your skin of its natural oils. Look for sulfate-free and pH-balanced options.

Toner

- Why: Toner removes any remaining residue from cleansing, balances your skin's pH and prepares it to absorb other skincare products better.
- How to Use: After cleansing, pour a small amount onto a cotton pad or your palms and pat it onto your face. Let it absorb completely.
- Tips: For oily or acne-prone skin, use toner with salicylic acid or witch hazel. For dry or sensitive skin, use hydrating toners with glycerin or aloe vera.

Antioxidants

- Why: Antioxidants defend your skin from free radicals caused by UV rays and pollution that can cause premature aging and dullness. They also brighten and even out your skin tone.
- How to Use: Apply 2-3 drops of a serum with vitamin C, green tea extract or ferulic acid onto your fingertips. Press it onto your skin.
- Tips: Vitamin C serums are best used in the morning and should be stored in a cool, dark place to prevent oxidation.

Moisturizer

- Why: Hydration is important even for oily skin. A good moisturizer locks in hydration and prevents dryness throughout the day.
- How to Use: Take a pea-sized amount and apply all over your face and neck. Focus on areas that tend to dry out.
- Tips: Use a lightweight, gel-based moisturizer if you have oily skin and a cream-based one for dry skin. Look for added benefits like niacinamide or ceramides for extra nutrition.

Sunscreen

- Why: Sunscreen is crucial for protecting your skin from harmful UV rays that can cause sunburn, premature aging and increase risk of skin cancer.
- How to Use: Apply a broad-spectrum SPF 30+ sunscreen all over your face and neck, at least 15 minutes before sun exposure. Reapply every 2 hours if outdoors.
- Tips: Look for non-comedogenic formulas to avoid clogged pores. If you wear makeup, try a tinted sunscreen or a lightweight formula that layers well under foundation.

Evening Routine

Cleanser

- Use a gentle cleanser. This will help remove any dirt, oil, and makeup that has accumulated throughout the day, leaving your skin feeling refreshed and clean.

Niacinamide Serum

- Improves skin texture, reduces the appearance of pores and blemishes, and brightens skin tone.

Night Cream

- Seals in the goodness, repairs and rejuvenates skin while you sleep

Other considerations, if you have oily skin, you might use a foaming cleanser and a lightweight, oil-free moisturizer. If you have dry skin, you might use a creamy cleanser and a rich, hydrating moisturizer. The key is to listen to your skin and adjust as needed. Consistency is key; a routine followed daily will give you better results over time.

In addition to these steps, you should also incorporate treatments and serums into your routine to address specific skincare concerns. These can be exfoliants, face masks and serums with active ingredients like vitamin C or alpha hydroxy acids. And don't forget to protect your skin from the sun by using a broad-spectrum sunscreen with at least SPF 30 daily, even on cloudy days.

Remember, consistency is key with skincare. Stick to your routine and give your skin time to adjust to the products. Don't be afraid to switch things up if something's not working for you and always listen to your skin.

Creating your personalized skincare routine may take some time and trial and error but the end result will be healthy, glowing skin you can be proud of. So, take the time to know your skin, choose the right products and stick to your routine for best results. Your skin will thank you.

6

Chapter 5: Glow Up

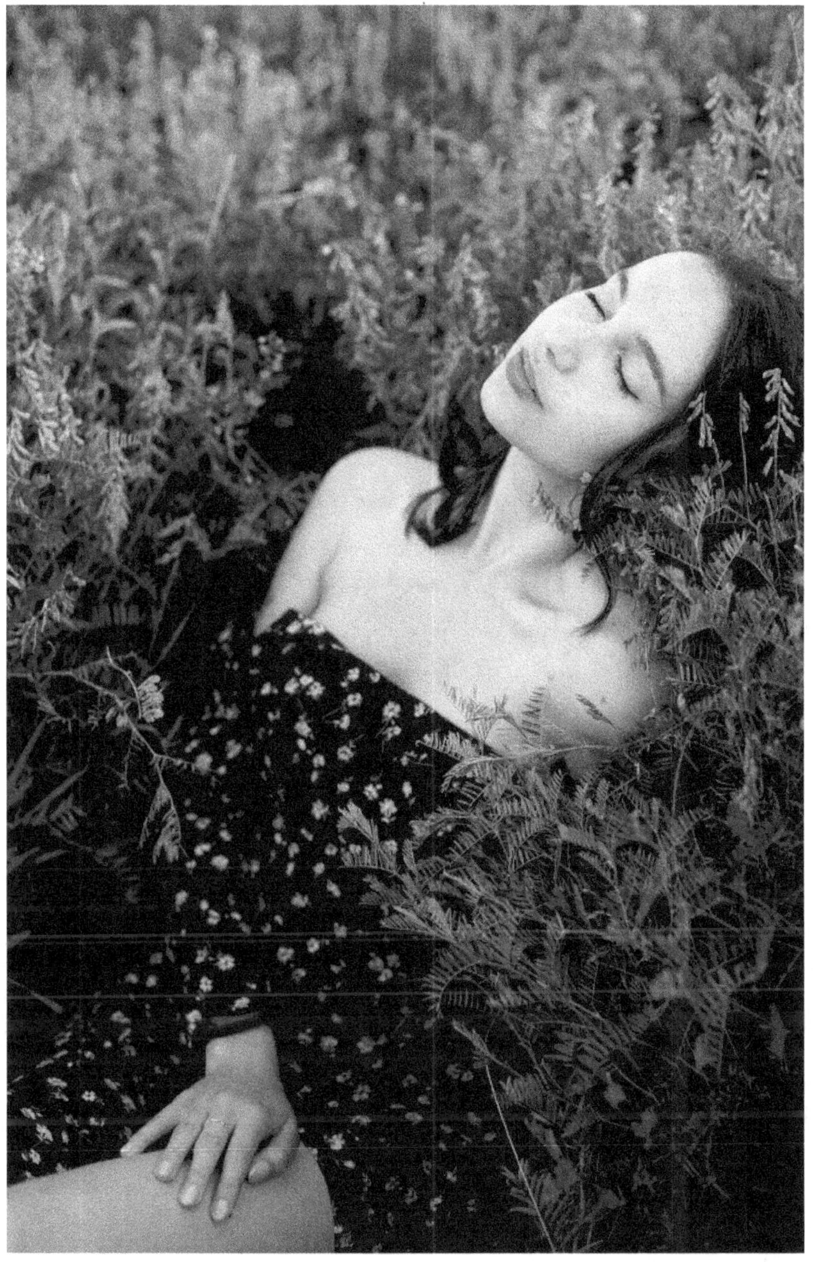

We are bombarded with images of airbrushed models and celebrities with perfect hair, flawless skin and "perfect" bodies. These unrealistic standards of beauty have been ingrained in us since we were young, making many of us feel insecure and inadequate.

But what if I told you true beauty is within you? What if I told you that embracing your own uniqueness is what makes you beautiful? It's time to redefine what beauty means and start living in a way that celebrates who we are, and glow up.

We all were born with features, characteristics and little details that make us unique. Those things aren't flaws—they're what make us stand out. Think about it—your freckles, your dimples, your laugh, your expressions—those are the things people love about you. Those are what make you memorable. Why do we spend so much time trying to erase or change them? Instead of trying to fit in with what society calls "beautiful" let's embrace the things that make us one of a kind. There's no one else out there like you and that's something to celebrate.

Redefining beauty isn't just about us; it's about changing the world's perspective. It's about creating space for everyone to feel seen and valued for who they are.

Imagine a world where we celebrate beauty in every shape, size, and color. Where we don't just tolerate differences—we embrace and honor them. Beauty isn't a "one size fits all" thing; it's a spectrum. The more we accept ourselves, the more we can encourage others to do the same. It's time to break free from the narrow definitions society has fed us and create new ones that are as diverse as we are.

Redefining beauty standards means breaking free from the limitations of society's narrow definition of beauty. It means celebrating diversity and inclusivity and that beauty comes in all shapes, sizes and colors. It's about accepting ourselves and others for who they are and not trying to fit into an unrealistic and unattainable standard.

And glowing up? It's about taking care of yourself in ways that matter. Feeding your body, mind, and soul what they truly need. This isn't about punishing yourself with diets or workouts you hate. It's about movement that makes you feel alive, eating in a way that energizes you, and finding time to rest and recharge. It's about saying no to the things that drain you and yes to the things that nourish you. When you take care of yourself, you feel better—and that inner peace and energy show up in ways no makeup or filter ever could.

It's time to stop chasing perfection and start living authentically. Let's create a world where beauty isn't about fitting in, but about standing out as yourself.

The truth is, perfection doesn't exist—and that's okay. What does exist is *you*, with all your unique qualities and potential. Let's stop striving for some unrealistic ideal and instead focus on being the best versions of ourselves. When we do, we not only feel better but also inspire others to embrace their true selves. So, let's redefine what it means to glow up—not to change who we are, but to fully embrace it.

7

Conclusion

I t is clear that our skin serves a bigger purpose than just simply being a surface of our body. It's a complex organ that plays a big role in our overall health and wellness. By knowing the secrets to glowing skin we can not only improve our physical appearance but also our overall quality of life.

Through proper skincare, healthy diet and positive mindset we can unlock our skin's full potential and get that glow. Remember beauty is not just skin deep but it also radiates from within. Taking care of our skin is not just about vanity but it's a form of self care and self love.

Let's glow-up our unique skin, flaws and all and treat it with kindness and nourishment it deserves. Because when we have healthy and glowing skin, we feel more confident and comfortable in our own skin. So, let's all strive to unlock the secrets to glowing skin and be our true beauty inside and out.

Glowing skin isn't a one size fits all formula. It's a personalized journey that combines science, care and a dash of patience. The journey beyond skincare is a transformative one where beauty is not just on the surface but a reflection of overall wellness. By embracing a holistic approach that includes nutrition, mindfulness and lifestyle changes you can unlock the secret to glowing skin. Remember beauty is a journey not a destination and it starts with self nurturing from the inside out.

Go! Glow!

Thank you for reading **Skin Deep: Unlocking the Secrets to Radiant Skin -** *A Guide to Skin Types, Skincare Ingredients and Creating Your Own Routines for Radiant Skin!* If you enjoyed the story, I'd be incredibly grateful if you could leave a review on Amazon. Your feedback not only helps me as an author but also helps other readers discover the book. Thank you for your support.

Resources

- *Paula's Choice Ingredient Dictionary: o Explains skincare ingredients and their benefits.* (n.d.). paulaschoice.com.
- Baumann, L. (2006). *The Skin Type Solution.* Fu And Lu, V. and G. (n.d.). *Skincare Decoded: o Practical and science-backed advice for crafting routines.*
- *Nature.* (2024, December 11). Nature. https://nature.com/
- *PubMed.* (n.d.). PubMed. https://pubmed.ncbi.nlm.nih.gov/

www.ingramcontent.com/pod-product-compliance
Lightning Source LLC
Chambersburg PA
CBHW071553260726
48653CB00008BA/3124